Healing Therapy
To Erectile Dysfunction
Impotence

By Taylor Jones

Introduction:

Erectile dysfunction ED, commonly referred to as impotence, is a prevalent and often underdiscussed medical condition that significantly affects the lives of countless men worldwide. This condition revolves around the inability to achieve or maintain a satisfactory erection during sexual activity, leading to a range of physical, emotional, and interpersonal challenges. The topic of erectile dysfunction holds immense importance not only for its impact on individual well-being but also for its implications on relationships, self-esteem, and overall quality of life.

**Importance's of discussing the topic
Erectile Dysfunction
Impotence**

Discussing the topic of Erectile Dysfunction Impotence is of paramount importance due to

its significant impact on both individual well-being and relationships. Here are key reasons why

discussing this topic is crucial:

1. **Health Awareness and Education:** Open discussions about erectile dysfunction contribute to raising awareness and educating individuals about the condition.

By understanding the causes, risk factors, and available treatment options, men can make informed decisions to manage their health effectively.

2. **De-stigmatization:** Talking openly about erectile dysfunction helps break down the stigma associated with it. Men often feel embarrassed or emasculated by the condition, which can prevent them from seeking necessary medical assistance. Creating an environment where ED is discussed openly promotes empathy and understanding, making it easier for affected individuals to seek help without shame.

3. **Timely Medical Intervention:** Early intervention is key to addressing erectile dysfunction effectively. Discussing the topic openly encourages men to consult healthcare professionals sooner, leading to timely diagnosis and appropriate treatment. Addressing the condition promptly can prevent its progression and associated complications.

4. **Relationship Enhancement:** Communication about erectile dysfunction within relationships is vital. Partners need to understand that ED is a medical issue and not a reflection of their desirability. Open conversations promote emotional closeness,

dispelling, misunderstandings and fostering support between partners during the treatment process.

5. **Improved Mental Health:** The psychological impact of erectile dysfunction can be significant, leading to feelings of inadequacy, anxiety, and depression. Openly addressing the topic helps men recognize that they are not alone in facing these challenges, potentially reducing feelings of isolation and improving mental well-being.

6. **Quality of Life Improvement:** Effective management of erectile dysfunction can lead to improved sexual function, higher self-esteem, and overall enhanced quality of life. By discussing the topic, individuals can access information about various treatment options that suit their needs and preferences.

7. **Prevention and Risk Reduction:** Discussing the risk factors for erectile dysfunction allows individuals to take proactive steps to prevent its development. Lifestyle changes such as maintaining a healthy diet, staying physically active, and avoiding tobacco and excessive alcohol consumption can significantly reduce the likelihood of experiencing ED.

8. **Advancement in Research:** Open conversations about erectile dysfunction can stimulate research efforts to further understand the condition's causes, mechanisms, and potential treatments.

This can lead to the development of more effective therapies and interventions.

Chapter 1

Definition of Erectile dysfunction

Erectile dysfunction ED, also commonly referred to as impotence, is a medical condition characterized by the consistent inability to achieve or maintain an erection sufficient for satisfactory sexual performance. This condition affects men of varying ages and can have profound physical, psychological, and relational implications. ED is not uncommon and can occur intermittently due to various factors, but when it becomes persistent and interferes with one's ability to engage in sexual activity and maintain healthy relationships, it warrants medical attention and intervention.

Physiology of Erection:

Erection is a complex physiological process that involves the integration of multiple systems within the body. When a man becomes sexually aroused, his brain sends signals to the nerves in the penis, triggering the release of neurotransmitters such as nitric oxide. Nitric oxide relaxes the smooth muscles within the blood vessels of the penis, causing them to dilate and allowing a higher volume of blood to flow into the erectile tissues known as the corpora cavernosa and corpus spongiosum. The increased blood flow engorges these tissues, leading to the expansion and hardening of the penis, resulting in an erection.

Chapter 2

Understanding erectile dysfunction

❖ **Physiology factors**

Certainly, the physiology of erection plays a crucial role in understanding erectile dysfunction. Here's a detailed overview of the physiology of erection and its connection to the topic of erectile dysfunction,

❖ **Physiology of Erection**

Erection is a complex physiological process that involves a coordinated interaction between the nervous, vascular, and endocrine systems. It begins with sexual arousal, which triggers a series of events that ultimately result in the engorgement and expansion of the erectile tissues in the penis.

1. **Sexual Arousal:** The process of erection begins with sexual stimulation, whether through physical touch,

visual cues, fantasies, or emotional triggers. This stimulation activates specialized nerve receptors

known as mechanoreceptors, which transmit signals to the brain's sexual centers.

2. **Neurotransmitter Release:** In response to sexual stimulation, the brain releases neurotransmitters that initiate a cascade of events. One of the key neurotransmitters involved is nitric oxide NO. Nitric oxide is released from nerve endings in the erectile tissues, including the corpus cavernosum and corpus spongiosum, which are sponge-like structures within the penis.

3. **Vasodilation:** Nitric oxide acts as a vasodilator, causing the blood vessels within the penis to relax and widen. This relaxation is particularly significant in the arterioles small arteries, that supply blood to the erectile tissues. As these blood vessels expand, they allow a higher volume of blood to flow into the penis.

4. **Increased Blood Flow:** The dilation of the blood vessels results in an increased inflow of blood into the erectile tissues.

This influx of blood engorges the corpus cavernosum and corpus spongiosum, causing them to expand and become firm.

5. **Trapping of Blood**: Simultaneously, the veins that normally carry blood away from the penis become compressed against the rigid outer shell of the erectile tissues. This compression prevents the outflow of blood, effectively trapping it within the erectile tissues and maintaining the erection.

6. **Nerve Stimulation**: The engorgement of the erectile tissue's places pressure on the surrounding nerves, contributing to the stimulation of sensory receptors. This stimulation generates pleasurable sensations and further enhances sexual arousal.

7. **Sustained Erection**: As long as sexual arousal continues and the signaling pathways remain active, the erection is maintained. Once sexual stimulation diminishes, the body's natural mechanisms allow the blood to flow out of the erectile tissues, leading to the gradual loss of erection.

Connection to Erectile Dysfunction:

Erectile dysfunction occurs when there is a disruption in any of the processes involved in achieving or maintaining an erection. Factors that can interfere with the physiology of erection include

A. Impaired Nitric Oxide Production: Conditions like diabetes, hypertension, and atherosclerosis can lead to reduced nitric oxide production, hampering the vasodilation necessary for an erection.

B. Vascular Issues: Narrowed or damaged blood vessels can restrict blood flow into the penis, preventing adequate engorgement of the erectile tissues.

C. Neurological Disorders: Nerve damage or conditions affecting the nervous system can disrupt the transmission of signals necessary for the erection process.

D. Psychological Factors: Anxiety, stress, depression, and performance anxiety can affect the brain's ability to initiate the release of neurotransmitters necessary for sexual arousal.

Understanding the intricate physiology of erection provides insights into the mechanisms that can go awry in cases of erectile dysfunction. Addressing these underlying issues through medical intervention, lifestyle changes, and psychological support can help restore normal erectile function and improve the overall quality of life for individuals experiencing ED.

❖ **Causes of Erectile Dysfunction:**

Certainly, the causes of erectile dysfunction ED, also known as impotence, are multifaceted and can involve a combination of physical, psychological, and lifestyle factors.

Erectile dysfunction can be attributed to a diverse range of causes, spanning both physical and psychological origins. Physical factors encompass conditions such as diabetes, cardiovascular diseases, hormonal imbalances, obesity, and certain medications. On the other hand, psychological factors, including stress, anxiety, depression, and performance anxiety, can contribute significantly to

the development and persistence of erectile dysfunction. Moreover, lifestyle choices like smoking, excessive alcohol consumption, and a sedentary routine can exacerbate the condition.

❖ **Physical Causes:**

1. **Vascular Conditions:** Cardiovascular diseases, such as atherosclerosis hardening of arteries, can lead to reduced blood flow to the penis, making it difficult to achieve and maintain an erection. Hypertension high blood pressure and high cholesterol levels can also contribute to vascular problems.

2. **Diabetes:** Diabetes can damage blood vessels and nerves, impairing the body's ability to transmit signals necessary for erection. Over time, poorly controlled diabetes can lead to nerve and blood vessel damage, exacerbating ED.

3. **Hormonal Imbalances:** Low levels of testosterone, the primary male sex hormone, can lead to reduced sexual desire and erectile difficulties.

Other hormonal imbalances, such as thyroid disorders, can also contribute to ED.

4. **Neurological Disorders:** Conditions like multiple sclerosis, Parkinson's disease, and spinal cord injuries can disrupt nerve signals responsible for initiating and maintaining an erection.

5. **Pelvic Surgery or Trauma:** Surgical procedures or injuries in the pelvic area, including those affecting the prostate, bladder, or spinal cord, can damage nerves and blood vessels critical for erectile function.

6. **Medications:** Some medications, including those used to treat hypertension, depression, anxiety, and certain prostate conditions, can have side effects that contribute to erectile dysfunction.

7. **Pyronine's Disease:** This condition involves the development of scar tissue within the penis, causing curvature and pain during erection, which can lead to ED.

8. **Obesity:** Excess body weight can contribute to hormonal imbalances, insulin resistance, and cardiovascular problems that negatively impact erectile function.

9. **Chronic Illnesses:** Conditions like kidney disease, liver disease, and chronic obstructive pulmonary disease COPD can lead to systemic changes that affect erectile function.

❖ **Psychological Causes:**

1. **Stress and Anxiety:** High levels of stress and anxiety, whether related to work, relationships, or other factors, can interfere with the brain's ability to initiate the processes that lead to sexual arousal and erection.

2. **Depression:** Depression affects neurotransmitter balance in the brain, including those involved in sexual arousal, potentially leading to reduced sexual desire and ED.

3. **Performance Anxiety**: Worrying about sexual performance and fearing failure can create a cycle of anxiety that inhibits the relaxation necessary for erection.

4. **Body Image Issues**: Negative body image or low self-esteem can lead to reduced sexual confidence and hinder sexual arousal.

❖ **Lifestyle Factors**

1. **Smoking**: Smoking damages blood vessels and reduces blood flow, contributing to vascular-related ED.

2. **Alcohol and Substance Abuse**: Excessive alcohol consumption and drug use can impair nerve function, decrease libido, and disrupt hormonal balance.

3. **Sedentary Lifestyle**: Lack of physical activity can contribute to obesity, cardiovascular problems, and hormonal imbalances that affect erectile function.

4. **Poor Diet**: A diet high in unhealthy fats, sugars, and processed foods can lead to obesity and other health conditions that impact ED.

5. **sleep disorders**: Conditions like sleep apnea can lead to reduced oxygen levels and affect overall health, including sexual function.

6. **Relationship Issues**: Poor communication, lack of emotional intimacy, and unresolved conflicts within relationships can contribute to ED.

7. **Age**: While aging itself isn't a cause of ED, older men are more likely to experience underlying health conditions that can contribute to erectile difficulties.

Addressing erectile dysfunction requires a comprehensive understanding of its causes, as treatment plans are tailored to the underlying factors. Consulting a healthcare professional is crucial for accurate diagnosis and appropriate management of this condition. In many cases, addressing lifestyle factors, managing underlying medical conditions, and seeking psychological support can significantly improve erectile function and overall quality of life.

❖ **Physical factors of Erectile dysfunction**

Certainly, physical factors play a significant role in the process of erection and can contribute to the development of erectile dysfunction. Here's an in-depth discussion of the physical factors involved:

❖ **Physical Factors Affecting Erection**

1. **Vascular Health**: Adequate blood flow to the penis is crucial for achieving and maintaining an erection. Conditions that affect blood vessels, such as atherosclerosis build-up of plaque in arteries, hypertension high blood pressure, and peripheral artery disease, can restrict blood flow to the penis, leading to erectile difficulties.

2. **Endocrine System**: Hormones, including testosterone, play a key role in sexual function. Low testosterone levels, a condition known as hypogonadism, can lead to reduced sexual desire and

difficulties in achieving and maintaining an erection.

3. **Neurological Factors**: Proper nerve function is essential for transmitting signals that initiate the physiological processes leading to an erection. Nerve damage or conditions that affect the nervous system, such as diabetes or spinal cord injuries, can disrupt these signals and lead to erectile dysfunction.

4. **Penile Structure and Health**: Conditions affecting the physical structure of the penis, such as Pyronine's disease formation of scar tissue or anatomical abnormalities, can cause pain during erection or curvature of the penis, leading to difficulties in achieving a firm and straight erection.

5. **Systemic Diseases**: Chronic diseases like diabetes, cardiovascular diseases, and kidney disease can contribute to erectile dysfunction by impairing blood vessel function, reducing nerve sensitivity, and causing hormonal imbalances.

6. **Medications**: Certain medications, including those used to treat high blood pressure, depression, anxiety, and prostate conditions, can have side effects that affect blood flow, nerve function, or hormone levels, contributing to erectile difficulties.

7. **Obesity**: Excess body weight is associated with hormonal imbalances, insulin resistance, and cardiovascular problems that can negatively impact erectile function.

8. **Substance Abuse**: Excessive alcohol consumption and drug use can lead to nerve damage, hormonal imbalances, and cardiovascular issues that contribute to ED.

9. **Pelvic Surgery or Trauma**: Surgical procedures or injuries in the pelvic region, such as those affecting the prostate, bladder, or spinal cord, can damage nerves and blood vessels necessary for achieving an erection.

❖ **Connection to Erectile Dysfunction**

These physical factors can lead to erectile dysfunction by interfering with the physiological processes that are essential for achieving and maintaining an erection. For example:

A. Vascular problems reduce blood flow to the penis, preventing proper engorgement of the erectile tissues.

B. Hormonal imbalances like low testosterone levels can lead to reduced sexual desire and difficulty in achieving an erection.

C. Nerve damage disrupts the transmission of signals necessary for initiating an erection.

D. Medications with side effects affecting blood flow, nerve function, or hormone levels can contribute to ED.

Addressing physical factors requires a holistic approach that may involve lifestyle changes, medical interventions, and consultation with healthcare professionals. Managing underlying health conditions, optimizing cardiovascular health, and maintaining a healthy lifestyle can significantly improve blood flow, nerve function, and hormonal balance, ultimately enhancing erectile function and overall sexual well-being.

❖ **Psychological factors**

Certainly, psychological factors play a significant role in the process of achieving and maintaining an erection, and they can contribute to the development of erectile dysfunction ED.

Here's a detailed discussion of the psychological factors involved:

❖ **Psychological Factors Affecting Erection**

1. **Stress and Anxiety**: High levels of stress and anxiety can trigger the release of stress hormones like cortisol, which can interfere with the body's ability to initiate and maintain an erection. Performance anxiety, particularly related to concerns about sexual performance and satisfying a partner, can create a cycle of worry that inhibits relaxation and arousal.

2. **Depression**: Depression is associated with altered brain chemistry, including imbalances in neurotransmitters like serotonin and dopamine. These imbalances can affect sexual desire, arousal, and the ability to achieve an erection.

3. **Performance Anxiety**: Fear of not being able to perform adequately during sexual activity can lead to anxiety, tension, and an inability to relax. This anxiety can disrupt the physiological processes necessary for an erection.

4. **Body Image Issues**: Negative body image and poor self-esteem can lead to a lack of sexual confidence and reduced ability to become sexually aroused.

5. **Relationship Issues**: Difficulties within intimate relationships, including communication problems, unresolved conflicts, or emotional distance, can create stress and emotional strain that impact sexual desire and function.

6. **Trauma and Past Experiences**: Previous traumatic sexual experiences, abuse, or emotional trauma can contribute to sexual anxiety and affect the ability to achieve or maintain an erection.

7. **Mental Health Conditions**: Conditions such as anxiety disorders, post-traumatic stress disorder PTSD, and obsessive-compulsive disorder OCD can lead to heightened stress levels that negatively impact sexual function.

8. **Negative Sexual Beliefs**: Cultural or societal messages, misconceptions about sex, or unrealistic expectations about sexual performance can create psychological barriers that hinder sexual arousal and function.

❖ **Connection to Erectile Dysfunction**

Psychological factors can significantly influence the process of achieving and maintaining an erection. For example:

A. Stress and anxiety trigger the release of stress hormones that can interfere with the body's ability to relax blood vessels and engorge the erectile tissues.

B. Depression alters neurotransmitter balance, affecting sexual desire and overall sexual function.

C. Performance anxiety can create a self-perpetuating cycle of stress and worry that impairs sexual arousal.

D. Negative body image and self-esteem can lead to reduced sexual confidence and difficulty in becoming sexually aroused.

Addressing psychological factors requires a comprehensive approach that may involve therapy, counseling, and lifestyle changes. Cognitive-behavioral therapy CBT and other forms of psychotherapy can help individuals manage anxiety, depression, and negative thought patterns related to sexual performance. Additionally, open communication within relationships and a supportive environment can mitigate the impact of psychological factors on sexual function. Consulting with a mental health professional or sex therapist can provide valuable guidance for addressing these psychological aspects of erectile dysfunction.

❖ **Lifestyle factors**

Certainly, lifestyle factors play a significant role in the development of erectile dysfunction ED. These factors can either contribute to or mitigate the risk of experiencing ED. Here's a detailed discussion of the lifestyle factors involved:

❖ **Lifestyle Factors Affecting Erection**

1. **Smoking**: Smoking damages blood vessels and reduces blood flow throughout the body, including to the penis. This can hinder the ability to achieve and maintain an erection.

2. **Alcohol Consumption**: Excessive alcohol intake can depress the central nervous system, dampen sexual desire, and impair nerve function. Chronic alcohol abuse can lead to long-term erectile difficulties.

3. **Drug Use**: Illicit drug use, particularly stimulants, depressants, and opioids, can negatively impact nerve function, hormonal balance, and overall sexual health.

4. **Physical Activity**: Regular exercise promotes cardiovascular health, improves blood flow, and helps maintain a healthy body weight. Sedentary behavior contributes to obesity and other health conditions that can affect erectile function.

5. **Diet**: A balanced diet rich in fruits, vegetables, lean proteins, and whole grains supports overall health, including cardiovascular health. A poor diet high in saturated fats, sugars, and processed foods can contribute to obesity and vascular problems.

6. **Obesity**: Excess body weight is linked to hormonal imbalances, insulin resistance, and cardiovascular issues that can impair erectile function.

7. **Sleep Quality**: Poor sleep patterns and sleep disorders can lead to hormonal imbalances, reduced energy levels, and overall health problems that contribute to ED.

8. **Stress Management**: Chronic stress triggers the release of stress hormones that can negatively impact the ability to achieve and maintain an erection. Practicing stress reduction techniques like mindfulness, yoga, and meditation can be beneficial.

❖ **Connection to Erectile Dysfunction**

Lifestyle factors can directly influence the physiological processes involved in achieving and maintaining an erection. For example:

A. Smoking damages blood vessels, leading to reduced blood flow to the penis.

B. Excessive alcohol intake depresses the central nervous system and dampens sexual desire.

C. Sedentary behavior contributes to obesity, which can lead to hormonal imbalances and cardiovascular problems.

D. Poor diet and obesity can negatively impact overall health, including the health of blood vessels and nerves necessary for an erection.

E. Chronic stress triggers the release of stress hormones that inhibit relaxation and arousal.

Addressing lifestyle factors often involves making positive changes to promote overall health and well-being. Engaging in regular physical activity, maintaining a balanced diet, avoiding smoking and excessive alcohol consumption, and managing stress effectively can have a positive impact on erectile function. Making healthier lifestyle choices can contribute not only to improved sexual health but also to enhanced overall quality of life. If lifestyle changes alone do not alleviate erectile dysfunction, seeking guidance from healthcare professionals is important to explore other potential causes and treatment options.

Chapter 3

Types of Erectile dysfunction

1. Organic Erectile Dysfunction

2. Psychogenic Erectile Dysfunction

3. Mixed/Combined Erectile Dysfunction

❖ **Organic Erectile dysfunction**

Certainly, "Organic Erectile Dysfunction" is a specific type of erectile dysfunction ED that arises primarily from physical or medical factors. It refers to cases where there is an identifiable physiological reason that disrupts the normal process of achieving and maintaining an erection. Here's a detailed explanation of organic erectile dysfunction:

❖ **Understanding Organic Erectile Dysfunction**

Organic erectile dysfunction, also known as organic impotence, occurs when there is an underlying physical cause that interferes with the complex

physiological processes required for an erection. Unlike psychogenic erectile dysfunction, which stems primarily from psychological factors, organic ED has a distinct physiological basis that can be identified through medical evaluation.

❖ **Causes of Organic Erectile Dysfunction**

Numerous physical factors can contribute to the development of organic erectile dysfunction. These factors can disrupt blood flow, nerve function, or hormonal balance, all of which are essential components of achieving and maintaining an erection. Some common causes include:

1. **Vascular Issues**: Conditions such as atherosclerosis plaque buildup in arteries, hypertension high blood pressure, and peripheral vascular disease can restrict blood flow to the penis, making it difficult to achieve and sustain an erection.

2. **Neurological Disorders**: Diseases that affect the nervous system, such as multiple sclerosis, Parkinson's disease, and spinal cord injuries, can disrupt nerve signals responsible for initiating and maintaining an erection.

3. **Endocrine Imbalances**: Hormonal imbalances, particularly low levels of testosterone, can lead to reduced sexual desire and difficulties in achieving an erection.

4. **Diabetes**: Uncontrolled diabetes can damage blood vessels and nerves, affecting the body's ability to transmit signals necessary for erection.

5. **Pelvic Surgery or Trauma**: Surgical procedures or injuries in the pelvic region, such as those affecting the prostate or bladder, can damage nerves and blood vessels necessary for erectile function.

6. **Medications**: Certain medications, including those used to treat high blood pressure, depression, and prostate conditions, can have side effects that contribute to ED.

7. **Pyronine's Disease**: This condition involves the development of scar tissue within the penis, causing curvature and pain during erection, which can lead to ED.

❖ **Diagnosis and Treatment**

Diagnosing organic erectile dysfunction involves a comprehensive medical evaluation. A healthcare professional will assess the individual's medical history, conduct physical examinations, and may recommend tests such as blood tests, imaging studies, and nerve function assessments. Identifying the underlying physical cause is crucial for devising an effective treatment plan.

Treatment of organic ED varies based on the specific cause. It may involve addressing underlying health conditions, such as managing diabetes or hypertension, hormone replacement therapy for testosterone deficiencies, or surgical interventions to correct anatomical issues. Lifestyle changes like adopting a healthier diet, engaging in regular

exercise, and quitting smoking can also contribute to improving vascular health and erectile function.

❖ **Psychogenic Erectile Dysfunction**

Certainly, "Psychogenic Erectile Dysfunction" is a specific type of erectile dysfunction ED that primarily arises from psychological or emotional factors. It refers to cases where psychological issues, rather than physiological factors, are the primary cause of difficulties in achieving and maintaining an erection.

Here's a detailed explanation of psychogenic erectile dysfunction:

❖ **Understanding Psychogenic Erectile Dysfunction:**

Psychogenic erectile dysfunction, also known as psychogenic impotence, occurs when psychological or emotional factors play a significant role in the inability to achieve or sustain an erection. Unlike organic erectile dysfunction, which stems primarily from physical factors, psychogenic ED has its basis in the mind and emotions.

❖ **Causes of Psychogenic Erectile Dysfunction:**

Several psychological factors can contribute to the development of psychogenic erectile dysfunction. These factors can create mental and emotional barriers that interfere with the complex neurological and physiological processes required for sexual arousal and erection. Some common causes include:

1. **Anxiety and Stress**: High levels of anxiety and stress, whether related to performance, work, relationships, or other issues, can lead to the release of stress hormones that inhibit the brain's ability to initiate the processes that lead to sexual arousal and erection.

2. **Depression**: Depression can alter neurotransmitter balance in the brain, including serotonin and dopamine, which play a role in sexual desire and overall sexual function.

3. **Performance Anxiety**: Worrying about sexual performance and fearing failure can create a cycle of

anxiety that inhibits relaxation and arousal, making it difficult to achieve and maintain an erection.

4. **Body Image Issues**: Negative body image, low self-esteem, and feelings of inadequacy can create psychological barriers that impact sexual confidence and the ability to become aroused.

5. **Relationship Issues**: Difficulties within intimate relationships, including poor communication, unresolved conflicts, or emotional distance, can contribute to stress and emotional strain that negatively affect sexual desire and function.

6. **Past Trauma or Abuse**: Previous traumatic sexual experiences, abuse, or emotional trauma can lead to sexual anxiety and difficulties in achieving or maintaining an erection.

❖ Diagnosis and Treatment

Diagnosing psychogenic erectile dysfunction involves a thorough psychological assessment in addition to a medical evaluation. A healthcare professional or mental health specialist may use psychological questionnaires and interviews to understand the emotional and mental factors contributing to the condition.

Treatment of psychogenic ED often involves addressing the underlying psychological issues through therapy and counseling. Cognitive-behavioral therapy CBT, psychotherapy, and sex therapy are common approaches used to help individuals manage anxiety, depression, and performance-related worries. Open communication with a partner can also play a crucial role in overcoming psychogenic ED and building emotional intimacy.

❖ Mixed/Combined Erectile Dysfunction

Certainly, "Mixed/Combined Erectile Dysfunction" is a specific classification of erectile dysfunction ED that encompasses both physical and psychological factors as contributing causes. It refers to cases where an individual experiences difficulty in achieving and maintaining an erection due to a combination of physiological and emotional factors. Here's a detailed explanation of mixed/combined erectile dysfunction:

❖ Understanding Mixed/Combined Erectile Dysfunction

Mixed or combined erectile dysfunction refers to a situation where both physical and psychological factors contribute to the development of erectile difficulties. This classification recognizes that erectile dysfunction can often be a complex interplay between physiological and emotional aspects, and it acknowledges that both sets of factors can interact and exacerbate each other.

❖ Causes of Mixed/Combined Erectile Dysfunction:

The causes of mixed/combined erectile dysfunction are multifaceted, involving a combination of physical and psychological factors. Some common scenarios include:

1. **Vascular Health and Anxiety**: A person with existing vascular problems, such as high blood pressure or atherosclerosis, might develop anxiety about their ability to achieve an erection due to past experiences of failure. This anxiety can further exacerbate the vascular issues by releasing stress hormones that restrict blood flow.

2. Diabetes and Performance Anxiety: Individuals with diabetes, which affects nerve function and blood vessels, might develop performance anxiety due to past experiences of ED. This anxiety can, in turn, hinder the body's ability to initiate and sustain an erection.

3. Hormonal Imbalances and Depression: Hormonal imbalances, such as low testosterone, can contribute to reduced sexual desire and difficulties in achieving an erection. This hormonal imbalance might also lead to feelings of depression, further impacting overall sexual function.

4. Body Image Issues and Medication Side Effects: Negative body image can lead to psychological barriers that impact sexual confidence. Additionally, certain medications used to manage other health conditions might have side effects that contribute to erectile difficulties.

5. Chronic Illness and Relationship Strain: A chronic illness, such as kidney disease, can lead to both physical and emotional challenges. The stress of dealing with the illness might strain the individual's relationship, creating additional psychological barriers to achieving an erection.

❖ **Diagnosis and Treatment**

Diagnosing mixed/combined erectile dysfunction requires a comprehensive assessment that addresses both physical and psychological aspects. A healthcare professional will consider medical history, conduct physical examinations, and may use psychological assessments to identify underlying factors.

Treatment of mixed/combined ED involves a holistic approach that targets both the physiological and emotional aspects. This may involve addressing underlying health conditions, such as managing diabetes or hypertension, while also exploring psychological interventions like cognitive-behavioral therapy CBT to manage anxiety and depression.

Chapter 4

Risk factors

Certainly, here's a summary of the risk factors associated with erectile dysfunction:

❖ **Risk Factors of Erectile Dysfunction**

1. Age: The risk of erectile dysfunction increases with age, but it's not an inevitable consequence of getting older.

2. **Vascular Health**: Conditions that affect blood flow, such as atherosclerosis, hypertension, and high cholesterol, can contribute to ED.

3. **Diabetes**: Uncontrolled diabetes can damage blood vessels and nerves, leading to erectile difficulties.

4. **Hormonal Imbalances**: Low testosterone levels and other hormonal imbalances can impact sexual desire and function.

5. **Neurological Disorders**: Conditions like multiple sclerosis, Parkinson's disease, and spinal cord injuries can disrupt nerve signals involved in erection.

6. **Medications**: Some medications, particularly those used for hypertension, depression, and prostate conditions, can have side effects that affect erectile function.

7. **Psychological Factors**: Stress, anxiety, depression, performance anxiety, and relationship issues can contribute to ED.

8. **Obesity**: Excess body weight is linked to hormonal imbalances, cardiovascular problems, and reduced blood flow, all of which can affect erectile function.

9. **Smoking and Substance Abuse**: Smoking damages blood vessels, while excessive alcohol and drug use can impair nerve function and overall health.

10. **Sedentary Lifestyle**: Lack of physical activity contributes to obesity and cardiovascular issues that impact sexual health.

11. **Poor Diet**: Unhealthy eating habits can lead to obesity and other health conditions that affect erectile function.

12. **sleep disorders**: Poor sleep patterns and sleep apnea can lead to hormonal imbalances and overall health problems that contribute to ED.

13. **Relationship Issues**: Poor communication, unresolved conflicts, and emotional distance within relationships can impact sexual desire and function.

Addressing these risk factors through lifestyle changes, medical interventions, and psychological support can contribute to preventing or managing erectile dysfunction and improving overall sexual well-being.

Chapter 5

Diagnosis of Erectile dysfunction

Diagnosing erectile dysfunction ED involves a comprehensive process that aims to identify the underlying factors contributing to the condition. It typically requires a combination of medical evaluation, psychological assessment, and a detailed discussion of the individual's medical history and lifestyle. Here's a detailed overview of the diagnosis of erectile dysfunction:

❖ **Medical History**

A thorough medical history is essential to understand the context and potential causes of ED. The healthcare provider will ask questions about the following:

A. Onset and duration of the problem

B. Frequency and nature of difficulties in achieving or maintaining an erection

C. Any sudden or gradual changes in sexual function

D. Presence of any underlying medical conditions diabetes, cardiovascular disease, hormonal imbalances

E. History of surgeries, injuries, or trauma to the genital or pelvic area

F. Current medications, including prescription and over-the-counter drugs

❖ **Physical Examination**

A physical examination helps identify any anatomical or physical factors contributing to ED. This may involve:

A. Examination of the penis and testicles for any abnormalities, deformities, or signs of Pyronine's disease (scar tissue)

B. Assessment of cardiovascular health, including blood pressure measurement and examination of the blood vessels for signs of atherosclerosis or circulation issues

C. Examination of secondary sexual characteristics and overall physical health

❖ **Psychological Assessment**

Since psychological factors can contribute to ED, a psychological assessment is often included. This involves discussing emotional well-being, relationship dynamics, and any mental health conditions that might impact sexual function, such as anxiety or depression.

❖ **Laboratory Tests**

Laboratory tests may be ordered to assess hormonal levels, blood sugar, cholesterol, and other factors that could contribute to ED. These tests may include:

A. Blood tests to check hormone levels, including testosterone

B. Blood glucose level measurement to assess diabetes risk

C. Lipid profile to assess cholesterol levels and cardiovascular health

❖ **Imaging and Other Tests**

In some cases, additional tests might be required to further evaluate blood flow and identify any physical abnormalities. These tests may include:

A. Duplex ultrasound: This test evaluates blood flow to the penis by using sound waves to create images of blood vessels.

B. **Nocturnal penile tumescence NPT test**: This test measures erectile function during sleep and helps differentiate between physical and psychological causes of ED.

C. **Injection test**: A medication is injected into the penis to stimulate an erection, helping to determine if the issue is vascular in nature.

❖ **Psychological Evaluation**

For cases where psychological factors are suspected to be significant contributors, a thorough psychological evaluation may be recommended. This involves assessing mental health, relationship dynamics, and any history of trauma or abuse that might affect sexual function.

❖ **Combined Approach**

Since ED often has multiple contributing factors, a holistic approach involving both medical and psychological evaluation is crucial for accurate diagnosis. The healthcare provider will analyze the information gathered from various sources to identify the primary and secondary factors contributing to ED.

Once a comprehensive evaluation is completed, the healthcare provider can provide a diagnosis and recommend appropriate treatment options tailored to the individual's specific needs. A personalized treatment plan might involve lifestyle changes, medical interventions, psychological therapy, or a

combination of approaches to address the underlying causes of erectile dysfunction.

Chapter 6

Treatment options

Certainly, the treatment options for erectile dysfunction ED are diverse and depend on the underlying causes, the severity of the condition, and the individual's overall health. Treatment aims to address both physical and psychological factors contributing to ED. Here's a detailed overview of the treatment options for erectile dysfunction:

Lifestyle Changes

Healthy Diet: Adopting a balanced diet rich in fruits, vegetables, whole grains, lean proteins, and healthy fats can improve cardiovascular health and overall blood circulation.

Regular Exercise: Engaging in regular physical activity improves blood flow, helps manage weight, and promotes general health, all of which positively impact erectile function.

Quitting Smoking: Quitting smoking helps restore blood vessel health and enhances overall cardiovascular function.

Limiting Alcohol and Drug Use: Reducing alcohol intake and avoiding recreational drug use can improve nerve function and hormone balance.

Stress Management: Engaging in stress-reduction techniques such as mindfulness, meditation, and yoga can help alleviate psychological factors contributing to ED.

❖ **Psychological Interventions**

Counseling and Therapy: Cognitive-behavioral therapy CBT, sex therapy, and couples therapy can address anxiety, depression, and relationship issues that contribute to ED.

Stress Reduction: Techniques like relaxation exercises and mindfulness meditation can help manage stress and anxiety.

❖ **Medications**

Phosphodiesterase Type 5 PDE5 Inhibitors: Drugs like sildenafil Viagra, tadalafil Cialis, and vardenafil Levitra enhance blood flow to the penis by increasing the effects of nitric oxide, which relaxes blood vessels and helps achieve and maintain an erection.

Alprostadil: Available in various forms injection, suppository, cream, alprostadil helps widen blood vessels and increase blood flow to the penis.

Testosterone Replacement Therapy: For men with low testosterone levels, hormone replacement therapy can help improve sexual desire and erectile function.

Vacuum Erection Devices VEDs:

These mechanical devices create a vacuum around the penis, drawing blood into the erectile tissues to facilitate an erection. A constriction ring is then placed at the base of the penis to maintain the erection.

Penile Implants:

Surgical options include penile implants, which are devices implanted into the penis to facilitate erections. There are inflatable and semi-rigid implants available.

❖   **Lifestyle Medications:**

Bremelanotide Vyleesi: This medication helps stimulate sexual desire in women and can also be used off-label for men with psychological ED.

Dehydroepiandrosterone: DHEA is a hormone supplement that might help with ED, particularly in men with low testosterone levels.

Alternative and Herbal Remedies:

Some individuals explore herbal supplements like ginseng, L-arginine, and ginkgo biloba. However, the efficacy and safety of these options vary, and consulting a healthcare professional is essential.

❖   **Surgery**

Vascular Surgery: In cases where blood vessel issues are identified, surgical procedures can be performed to improve blood flow to the penis.

Penile Implants: As mentioned earlier, these devices can be surgically implanted to provide on-demand erections.

❖ **Combination Therapies**

Depending on the individual's specific situation, a combination of treatments might be recommended to address multiple contributing factors simultaneously.

❖ **Psychological Support:**

Sex Therapy: With the guidance of a sex therapist, individuals and couples can work through emotional barriers and improve communication related to sexual concerns.

Couples Counseling: Addressing relationship issues can enhance intimacy and alleviate performance anxiety.

❖ **Other treatment options**
❖ **For erectile dysfunction**

In addition to phosphodiesterase type 5 PDE5 inhibitors like sildenafil Viagra, tadalafil Cialis, and vardenafil Levitra, there are other medications that are being explored or used off-label for the treatment of erectile dysfunction ED. These medications target various aspects of the physiological process involved in achieving and maintaining an erection. Here's a detailed discussion of some of these alternative medications:

1. Bremelanotide Vyleesi:

Bremelanotide is a medication that stimulates sexual desire and arousal. It works by activating melanocortin receptors in the brain, which play a role in sexual motivation. Originally developed as a treatment for female sexual dysfunction, bremelanotide has also been studied and used off-label for men with psychological ED.

2. Dehydroepiandrosterone:

DHEA is a hormone produced by the adrenal glands that is a precursor to both testosterone and estrogen. Some research suggests that DHEA supplementation might help improve erectile function, especially in men with low testosterone levels. However, its effectiveness and safety for this purpose are still under investigation.

3. PDE5 Inhibitor Combinations:

Combining different PDE5 inhibitors or combining PDE5 inhibitors with other medications is an approach being explored to enhance their effectiveness in treating ED. This approach may be beneficial for individuals who don't respond well to single PDE5 inhibitors.

4. Melanocortin Receptor Agonists:

In addition to bremelanotide, other medications that target melanocortin receptors in the brain are being studied for their potential to enhance sexual desire and arousal. These medications could offer an alternative approach for individuals with psychological causes of ED.

5. Topical Medications:

Topical creams and gels containing specific medications, such as alprostadil or sildenafil, are being investigated as potential treatments for ED. These medications are applied directly to the penis and aim to improve blood flow and facilitate an erection.

6. L-arginine:

L-arginine is an amino acid that the body uses to produce nitric oxide, a molecule that helps relax blood vessels and improve blood flow. Some studies suggest that L-arginine supplements might help improve erectile function, although the evidence is mixed.

7. Herbal and Nutraceutical Supplements:

Certain herbal supplements, such as ginseng, ginkgo biloba, and maca root, are believed to have potential benefits for erectile function. However, the efficacy and safety of these supplements vary, and more research is needed to determine their effectiveness.

8. Future Developments:

Research is ongoing to explore new medications that target novel pathways involved in erectile function. As our understanding of the physiological processes involved in ED continues to evolve, new medications with innovative mechanisms of action may emerge.

It's important to note that not all of these medications have been thoroughly studied for their effectiveness and safety in treating ED. If considering any alternative medication or supplement, individuals should consult a healthcare professional to discuss potential risks, benefits, and interactions with other medications they may be taking. Additionally, off-label use of medications

should be approached with caution and under the guidance of a qualified healthcare provider.

Chapter 7

Prevention of Erectile dysfunction

Preventing erectile dysfunction ED involves a combination of maintaining overall health, managing risk factors, and adopting a healthy lifestyle. While not all cases of ED can be prevented, these measures can significantly reduce the likelihood of developing the condition. Here's a detailed overview of the prevention strategies for erectile dysfunction:

❖ **Maintain a Healthy Lifestyle**

Balanced Diet: Eat a diet rich in fruits, vegetables, whole grains, lean proteins, and healthy fats. Limit saturated fats, sugars, and processed foods.

Regular Exercise: Engage in regular physical activity to improve cardiovascular health, maintain a healthy weight, and enhance blood circulation.

Hydration: Drink plenty of water to maintain proper blood flow and overall health.

Avoid Smoking: Quit smoking or avoid starting altogether. Smoking damages blood vessels, reducing blood flow to the penis.

Moderate Alcohol Intake: Limit alcohol consumption to a moderate level, as excessive drinking can impair nerve function and hormone balance.

❖ **Manage Underlying Health Conditions**

Control Diabetes: Manage blood sugar levels effectively to prevent nerve and blood vessel damage.

Maintain Cardiovascular Health: Control blood pressure and cholesterol levels through a healthy lifestyle, medications, or a combination of both.

Hormonal Balance: If you suspect low testosterone levels, consult a healthcare professional to determine appropriate treatment options.

❖ **Prioritize Psychological Health**

Stress Management: Practice stress-reduction techniques such as mindfulness, meditation, yoga, and deep breathing exercises.

Healthy Relationships: Foster open communication and emotional intimacy with your partner to prevent stress and relationship-related ED.

Seek Counseling: Address mental health issues like anxiety, depression, or past trauma through counseling or therapy.

❖ **Limit Medications That Can Cause ED**

Consult a doctor: If you're taking medications that might contribute to ED, consult your doctor to explore alternative options or adjust dosages.

❖ Maintaing Regular Medical Checkups

Routine Checkups: Regularly visit a healthcare provider for checkups to monitor your overall health and address any emerging concerns.

❖ Avoid Illicit Drug Use

Recreational Drugs: Avoid or limit the use of recreational drugs, as they can negatively impact nerve function, hormonal balance, and overall health.

❖ Manage Obesity

Healthy Weight: Maintain a healthy weight through a balanced diet and regular exercise, as obesity is linked to various risk factors for ED.

Practice Safe Sex

Use Protection: Engage in safe sexual practices to prevent sexually transmitted infections STIs that could contribute to ED.

❖ Communication and Education

Open Dialogue: Talk openly with your partner about sexual health concerns and seek information to address any misconceptions.

❖ impacts of erectile dysfunction

Erectile dysfunction ED can have profound emotional and relationship impacts on individuals and their partners. The experience of ED goes beyond the physical aspect, affecting self-esteem, confidence, and intimacy. Here's a detailed discussion of the emotional and relationship impacts of erectile dysfunction:

❖ Emotional Impact

1. **Self-Esteem and Confidence**: ED can significantly lower self-esteem and erode confidence. Men may feel inadequate, less masculine, and question their worthiness as a partner.

2. **Anxiety and Stress**: The fear of experiencing ED during sexual encounters can lead to performance anxiety and heightened stress levels. This anxiety, in turn, can exacerbate the ED, creating a self-perpetuating cycle.

3. **Depression**: ED can contribute to feelings of sadness, hopelessness, and frustration. The inability to engage in a satisfying sexual relationship can trigger or worsen symptoms of depression.

4. **Guilt and Shame**: Men may feel guilty for not being able to satisfy their partners and may experience shame about their inability to perform sexually.

5. **Isolation**: Some men may withdraw socially and emotionally, avoiding intimacy altogether to prevent the possibility of facing ED.

6. **Loss of Identity**: For some, their self-identity may be closely tied to their sexual performance, and ED can challenge their sense of self.

❖ **Relationship Impact**

1. **Communication Breakdown**: The difficulty of discussing ED may lead to a breakdown in communication between partners. Open dialogue is essential for mutual understanding and finding solutions.

2. **Intimacy Issues**: ED can strain emotional intimacy as partners may become hesitant or fearful of engaging in sexual activities.

3. **Misinterpretation**: Partners might mistakenly assume that the lack of sexual interest or the inability to perform indicates a lack of attraction or love.

4. **Resentment and Frustration**: Partners may feel frustrated due to unfulfilled sexual needs and may even harbor resentment if they perceive their needs aren't being considered.

5. **Pressure and Expectations**: The pressure to perform sexually can create tension in the relationship, further exacerbating the ED. Unrealistic expectations contribute to this pressure.

6. **Loss of Connection**: The physical and emotional disconnection resulting from ED can weaken the bond between partners, leading to feelings of isolation and loneliness.

❖ **Coping Strategies:**

1. **Open Communication**: Talking openly about ED is crucial. Both partners should feel comfortable discussing their feelings, concerns, and needs.

2. **Seek Professional Help**: Consulting healthcare professionals and therapists can provide guidance, education, and strategies to manage the emotional and relationship impacts of ED.

3. **Explore Non-Sexual Intimacy**: Focus on building emotional connection through non-sexual activities, like spending quality time together and engaging in open conversations.

4. **Mutual Support**: Partners can offer empathy, understanding, and encouragement to each other, reinforcing their emotional bond.

5. **Education**: Learning about the causes and treatments of ED can demystify the condition and reduce stigma, fostering a more supportive environment.

6. **Professional Therapy**: Couples therapy can provide a safe space to address ED-related concerns, enhance communication, and work together to find solutions.

❖   **Future research and developments in the field of erectile dysfunction ED**

are aimed at expanding our understanding of the underlying causes, improving diagnostic methods, and advancing treatment options. Here's a detailed discussion of the potential areas of research and developments for ED:

1. Precision Medicine and Personalized Treatments

Future research might focus on identifying genetic, hormonal, and physiological factors that contribute to ED. This could lead to more personalized treatment approaches tailored to an individual's specific genetic and physiological makeup.

2. Neurological Advances:

Research into the neurological mechanisms involved in achieving and maintaining an erection could lead to innovative treatments targeting nerve signaling and pathways. This could be especially beneficial for individuals with neurogenic causes of ED.

3. Gene Therapy:

Gene therapy holds promise for addressing underlying causes of ED by introducing specific genes to enhance blood flow, nerve function, or hormonal balance.

4. Stem Cell Therapy:

Stem cell research might lead to the development of regenerative therapies that repair damaged blood vessels, nerves, and tissues involved in erectile function.

5. Advanced Imaging Techniques:

Improved imaging methods could provide real-time visualization of blood flow and changes in the erectile tissues during sexual arousal, enhancing our understanding of the physiological processes involved.

6. Non-Invasive Treatments:

Developments in non-invasive treatments like shockwave therapy and electromagnetic field therapy could offer alternative options for enhancing blood flow and promoting tissue regeneration.

7. Virtual Reality and Telemedicine:

Incorporating virtual reality and telemedicine into treatment could improve access to therapy, allowing individuals to receive counseling and treatment remotely.

8. Targeting Inflammation:

Exploring the role of chronic inflammation in ED could lead to therapies that target and reduce inflammation to improve erectile function.

9. Nutraceuticals and Supplements:

Research into the potential benefits of specific nutraceuticals, supplements, and herbal remedies might yield alternative or adjunctive treatments for ED.

10. Behavioral Interventions:

Research into behavioral interventions, such as mindfulness-based therapies, could provide non-pharmacological options for managing stress, anxiety, and depression that contribute to ED.

11. Psychological Interventions:

Advancements in understanding the psychological factors behind ED could lead to more effective therapies for managing performance anxiety, relationship issues, and other emotional barriers.

12. Combination Therapies:

Research might explore the effectiveness of combining multiple treatment modalities, such as medications, lifestyle changes, and psychological interventions, to address various contributing factors.

13. Long-Term Safety and Efficacy:

Continued research is crucial for evaluating the long-term safety and efficacy of existing and emerging treatments, ensuring that they remain effective and safe over time.

14. Public Awareness and Education:

Promoting public awareness and education about ED can help reduce stigma, encourage early intervention, and facilitate more open discussions about sexual health.

15. Patient-reported Outcomes:

Research on patient-reported outcomes can provide insights into the quality of life and overall well-being of individuals living with ED, informing treatment strategies and improvements.

Conclusion

Future research and developments in the field of erectile dysfunction hold the potential to revolutionize our understanding and management of the condition. Advances in genetics, neurology, regenerative medicine, and psychological interventions could offer more effective and personalized treatment options, ultimately improving the quality of life for individuals affected

by ED. Continued collaboration between medical professionals, researchers, and individuals with ED is essential to driving these advancements forward.

In conclusion, erectile dysfunction ED is a complex and multifaceted condition that can impact men of all ages. It goes beyond the physical aspect, affecting emotional well-being, relationships, and overall quality of life. While ED can stem from a combination of physiological and psychological factors, it's important to recognize that it's a treatable condition.

Advancements in medical research, diagnostics, and treatments have provided a range of options for addressing ED. From lifestyle changes and medications to psychological interventions and innovative therapies, there are tailored approaches to suit individual needs. Open communication between partners and with healthcare professionals is crucial for effective diagnosis and treatment.

Breaking down stigmas surrounding ED and promoting public awareness are vital steps towards encouraging early intervention and seeking

appropriate help. Understanding that ED is not a reflection of masculinity or self-worth, but rather a medical condition with various contributing factors, is pivotal in supporting those affected.

As we continue to progress in research and medical technology, the future holds promising developments that will further refine our understanding of ED and enhance treatment outcomes. The key lies in recognizing that seeking help is a sign of strength, and with the right support and guidance, individuals can regain control of their sexual health and overall well-being.